CW00848376

The Sapphire Conspiracy and beyond it all

By
Samantha Glynn

Copyright © 2017 Samantha Glynn

First Published 2017

The rights of the author have been asserted in accordance
with the Copyright, Designs and Patents Act 1988.

All rights reserved.
No part of this publication may be reproduced or
transmitted or utilized in any form or by any means,
electronic or mechanical, including photocopy, recording, or
any information storage and retrieval system without
permission in writing from the author.

ISBN-13:
978-1974542994

ISBN-10:
1974542998

Acknowledgements

I would like to thank all my friends and family that have helped me through this difficult time, and beyond. I mustn't forget those who didn't know me but helped me in hospital and during my recovery. I have described how many of you have helped me in this book.

I'd also like to thank my sister, Charlotte Dooley, for producing the artwork for the front cover. My dad for reading my book when my husband couldn't as it hurt too much to relive it all. My mum for her words of encouragement.

I would also like to thank my work colleagues who face similar difficulties day in and day out.

I have self-published this book and I would not have been able to do this without the help of Helen Baggott and Kit Foster.

Introduction

This is the story of my battle with mental health. It is exactly how I experienced it. Looking back I can still remember how I felt at the time. I'm through the worst of it now and I have learned to recognise the warning signs.

So am I glad I went into teaching? Yes. Would I do it all again? No.

Are more people becoming aware of mental health issues? I hope so.

The first part of this book looks at how quickly I was taken into hospital and describes what I remember about my stay there and indeed how necessary it was. It also describes my relapse and points out possible reasons for my illness. I was aware that 1 in 4 of us suffer mental health problems but I never really thought it would be me.

The second part looks at a few years later, at a time when the whole world seemed to be going mad with people dressed up as clowns running around scaring people and people trying to ram cars to get insurance money. It was up to me to remain calm and to carry on in my job. My anxiety tablets were helping but I could feel anxiety running through my veins at some points. Living day by day helped, and talking things through with my colleagues. We were all in the same boat and surely things could only get better. There had been numerous cutbacks at my school which hadn't helped student behaviour and workload.

The final part looks at the detailed reasons for my poor mental health and the steps I could take to improve it. It was really good to get some answers and to look at self-help strategies.

PART 1
The Sapphire Conspiracy

Chapter 1
The event

Well let's start with that day in June 2011. A normal day or so it seemed. I hadn't been sleeping all that well. I was waking up early worrying about work even though I had finished for the summer. I asked my husband if he could help with the school run as my children's summer holiday hadn't started yet. But having to work shifts he was really no good in the mornings. So I got changed. I can't remember if I brushed my hair. Probably not! I drove my children to school and this is when the conspiracy theory started in my head. I was working it all out and came up with the conclusion that the government was involved and they were testing our marriage and going to reward us with something. My husband works in the police and has a stressful job and I had recently trained in teaching.

I saw my son's teacher at the gate; he had a pass around his neck and it was then that I decided that government agents were involved and they were wearing such passes. I saw my children into the gate for the last time in what would be two weeks.

Walking back to the car I saw someone I knew. There was a brief discussion about class photos then I said, 'I've got to get back to talk to my husband.' I'm not really sure how I managed to drive home but I did and screeched into the driveway. It was almost as though I had dropped off my children at school and could now let go.

Going into the house, I started to shout out to myself. 'Right, you can come out now!' I was expecting agents from work to come out and explain that I had been part of a test and that I had passed and everything was going to be alright. My husband came down and did not understand what I was doing. At this point I said I was going to bed and I remember lying there while he called Social Services for advice. He then went downstairs and I shouted, 'A drink would be nice!' I'd later discover that I had drunk lots of Pepsi before I became ill but I don't remember really. Later, my husband went out on his bike for a short while; his way of coping I guess.

I lay in bed unable to sleep and decided to go into town. For some reason I had it in my head that I should make myself look a bit mad and wearing my husband's shoes would help with the effect! So I left the house taking a back glance at my neighbour's house – as this was empty and I imagined agents inside the house watching our every move.

I walked into town shuffling in an almost mad manner. Once I got to the local Co-op I went to the customer services counter and asked to see the manager. A small man that I had recognized from the area seemed to be following me so I thought he was an agent too. Even *The Big Issue* seller came into question as I entered the store. The cashier organised for me to go to the back of the store and upstairs to see the manager with a Co-op rep. I thought it would be safe if they could ring the police for me and reach my husband. I seemed to think he was at work. The manager started to make the call and I said, 'Someone's spoken to you haven't they?' Believing she was in on it and I was in danger I left the store.

Goodness knows what they thought but they seem friendly enough when I go in there now. After leaving the Co-op, still thinking I was being followed, I walked up the high street to sit on a bench. I saw a policeman and waved to show him I was alright. After a while I walked home, I can't remember that part.

Once home I was at the window of the bedroom, looking for my husband. He came back and I went down to warn him that someone was in our house and we could be killed. He tried to get me back in the house. This freaked me out so I started to run up the road in my socks. He tried to persuade me to go back. I didn't run too far and kept looking back. I thought I saw him on the phone so I shouted out, 'You can tell my boss his book sucks,' which was a little strange as I hadn't read it yet. But I was convinced he was one of the agents that my husband was in contact with.

During our time out the front I had asked a passer-by to help, saying there were people in our house and I called out for the police. A neighbour did come out which was reassuring.

My husband managed to get me back into the porch and said he was going to call for help. Help did arrive in the form of two policemen. I said I'd make a cup of tea. I'd been meaning to make one all day and I still didn't manage it. I sat in the lounge and they asked me some questions. I can't really remember the questions or what my answers were. In the end I just said, 'Can't I go to A and E and have a drip or something?'

My husband agreed to follow in the car and he got me some shoes (this would become a code word later on). My socks had become blackened after running up the road in them earlier. The police arranged to take me to A and E and they helped me cross the road and into the car. It felt claustrophobic and scary but I was glad to be taken to hospital.

Chapter 2
A and E

I remember the journey pretty well and feeling a bit sick in the back of the car. The policemen were talking to each other and keeping a look out for my husband following. When we arrived they parked right outside and the driver got out, at this point I panicked and tried to get out of the police car by the window. I think I struggled with one of them. They managed to calm me down and get me into the A and E corridor. I sat down and luckily my husband arrived.

We had to wait a short while to see the doctor. By the time I was seen I was a physical and mental wreck. I nearly collapsed on the floor; all I wanted was a drip and a good rest. They took me to a cubical where I lay down. I don't really remember what time it was but I remember my husband checking his watch. He was concerned about who was going to pick up our children from school and he had phoned my parents in Essex.

Eventually a nurse came to see me and took blood samples. Even this I was suspicious of. I would lay back and listen to what was going on outside my cubical. I was convinced I heard a man's voice from work (I think I even saw him). I thought he was a baddy from the conspiracy and then I heard two girls' voices from work who I thought were on the good side and somehow they had won. I could hear their voices clearly and they were celebrating. It was all going to be alright. But in the next instance I had convinced myself that a bomb was involved and that the only people that would be left in the hospital would be me and my husband.

It would be surrounded by government agents.

My husband doesn't like talking about it much but he remembers me asking him what would happen if we killed ourselves. I kept wondering why my husband looked so puzzled and worried. I thought that he may be being contacted by someone involved in the conspiracy.

I remember going to see a doctor at one point and answering some questions. I think I answered them honestly but possibly not, as one patient I later met described it as being away with the fairies. I finally had some food in the form of sandwiches and crisps. We were moved around from bed to bed to wait for various tests. One test involved an ambulance ride to Canterbury.

I remember going on about my theory in the ambulance and naming goodies and baddies. It was dark outside by this point and a nurse was sitting next to me making notes. She looked vaguely familiar but I couldn't place her. When we arrived she looked upset by it all as though she was feeling guilty, almost as though she was a lawyer for my work. My husband was with me which was probably all that stopped me running off when we stopped.

I was taken to have a CT scan of my head. I remember they were worried that I would move and ruin the scan but I remembered to stay still. The others had all gone into a separate room to avoid the X-rays. They came out and said, 'Well done,' and then I was trolleyed back to the ambulance, joking with the ambulance staff about pensions. I don't remember the journey back to Accident and Emergency.

Once we were back a couple of people from Social Services talked to us. I remember trying to act normal and this seemed to work. But at that stage I was far from normal. Eventually my husband could not stay any longer so he went, telling me to get some rest and to stay in my bed area. I wasn't relaxed enough to sleep so after a while I went wandering.

At this point I should tell you that I had watched a couple of films in the days leading up to my illness when I was stressed about contracts at work. One of them about child abduction and children's bones being found on a property in America. I can't remember the title but it was later to have an effect on me.

Chapter 3
Near escape

A nurse came up to me and tried to get me back to my bed but I ended up in another room. I lay down but sleep was not going to happen. She gave me some pills but I didn't take them. I could hear what sounded like a radio and I could hear what I thought was a news report that a man had been found wandering without his shoes and that two children were missing. I remember thinking that my husband had gone looking for my boys. I didn't really believe that one or both of my boys could be dead but it started to become part of my conspiracy theory. In my head a competition had started. If my husband could win the steps we would get our boys back.

I decided to start wandering again and went into a room where there were patients in beds and relatives sitting with them around a group of computers. I leant against the desk with the computers and started to explain to people that I had seen a film. They didn't take me seriously and I remember some laughing. A nurse came up to me and asked who I was. She checked it all out on a computer.

Quickly I decided that I had to take myself to the mental hospital. I must state this was due to the film that I had watched and not down to any accurate self-diagnosis! I had no idea where the nearest mental hospital was but was going to start walking in my gown. I walked past the computers and tried to get out of the exit, I was stopped and so I tried to get into another room. Some hospital staff followed and got me out. There was a lot of equipment in there and they were relieved I hadn't touched anything. Security had been called and he soon came up to me by a doorway. He was quite old and in a white shirt. I told him he was a lawyer and he asked me where I was going. I said I was going to walk to the mental hospital. The two social workers/police arrived again and I said, 'I've been waiting for you two to come back.' At this point I have no further memories of A and E as I may have been sedated.

Chapter 4
Sapphire Ward

My next memory is coming out of A and E in the dark, being held by two nurses. I noticed a police car with someone I thought was from work inside. I muttered 'bitch' under my breath as I had her down as one of the baddies. They got me into the ambulance and I was being taken to a special unit in Medway Hospital. On the journey I kept asking if I would see my boys alive when I got there. They did their best to reassure me but one did not look sincere and I picked up on this. So for most of the journey I kept asking them things and talking about my theory (in between nearly dozing off). I occasionally looked out of the front window and saw we were on a motorway and it was now starting to get light. One of them said that I would be greeted by crowds when we got there.

We arrived at the hospital and it was dark and empty as far as I could tell. They took me up to the ward and I was offered food. I went to take some crisps but then thought this might also be a trick so moved on. I don't remember much of the first few days or nights there and the rules that should be followed which became clear later on.

The order of the next events becomes a bit muddled but there were four main things other than when my husband and mum came to visit.

The first was me, wandering around looking for my bed area. This did not please a lot of patients, as you can imagine. A couple of nurses found me and sat with me asking me to think of positive thoughts. They had some tablets and finally

I trusted them enough to take them, I think they used the code word 'shoe' that my husband had used with me. I did get to know the ward eventually. I remember trying to get into locked rooms, calling out names from my conspiracy theory. I looked into one room which I called the suicide room, for a moment I thought I had seen a male patient in it, which is impossible as they were in a separate ward next door.

The second was being in the lounge area and thinking about the contest that was going on for which my husband was trying to win our boys back and become head of my school. The contest went on and on with my imagination of a commentary. At one point it was getting close to an ending and I was in another room. I could hear a helicopter outside as if my husband was about to win the contest and take over as head. Then I saw another baddy from work; he was trying to get in the building to stop it all. An alarm went off and I was being locked in the lounge. I started dancing in celebration when I saw him leave. I would show that other teacher at my school that I could act.

One of the nurses said later that she thought I was acting when I came into the unit. Far from it; I was just way out of control. Clearly I believed that my husband had won the competition as when he came to visit and asked who I thought he was I said he was my head teacher. He was clearly confused by this but my mum could see I wasn't myself.

Another major memory was being rather rude to a nurse (I later apologised) as I thought she was another lawyer. She was filling out paperwork and I was calling her thick and that all lawyers were thick, which is not what I think in reality. After this verbal abuse I was taken to another room and examined. I was asked to get undressed to my underwear and was weighed. The doctor said I was not as bad as when I had arrived. I think I had lost a lot of weight. Talking of which, once I got more of an idea of what was going on I figured out you could order food and the puddings were great, they were things like sponge puddings.

I only had one real incident in the canteen. This was when I was talking during dinner and thought everyone was listening to me so I stuffed a paper tissue in my mouth to stop me talking. This was the only time that I worried my friend, a fellow patient in there. I keep in touch with her on Facebook and she is now a mental health nurse, which is great. She used to bring her guitar in and I used to love listening to her play.

There are also snippets of memory of my stay.

Before I started to get better I remember my room was behind the staff desk so I could hear them. One night I had it in my head that the kidnappers of my kids also had my dad, probably because I hadn't seen my dad yet. He later visited me in hospital. I imagined that my dad was in the car outside but he was going to be taken away. I could hear the car door and everything. I remember crying and saying out loud, 'Poor Dad, it's all my fault.' I must have drifted off to sleep after this.

Another night there was someone sitting in my room keeping an eye on me. I looked up and said, 'You don't have to stay here if you don't want to.' She kind of looked at me and grunted. I thought 'ah well' and tried to get some rest. It may have been something to do with me choosing not to take a couple of tablets and hiding them on my windowsill.

One day when we had been taken down to make some clay models I walked into the art room and the radio was on. I remember hearing about the conspiracy theory on the radio; it was clear as day to me. The nurse could tell I was bothered by the radio and calmly turned it off. I could then focus on my art work which helped. I had also started to read in hospital. I had started reading the Katie Price autobiography.

Last night I went out for a curry and one of my friends joked that I must have been ill if I was reading that! I would tear out bits that were relevant to me. I apologised for this later. Unfortunately I didn't keep the bits that I had torn out but I did keep some notes that I made in hospital that would later prove useful in explaining my illness.

Early on I remember being upset about all the toing and froing that smoking breaks caused. I didn't smoke but all the commotion in the ward set me off. Later I would find music was a good distraction. My husband had brought in my Nintendo DS, music player and some money for chocolate.

In the evenings I would sometimes walk very fast down the corridors listening to my music. I had a flashback about walking down the corridor in my underwear but I have no idea if this happened or not!

Once I started to get better I realised that the conspiracy theory was all in my head. I tried to write down exactly what the conspiracy theory was but I couldn't. All I know is that I believed in it so much when I was ill. I didn't really feel silly as I knew exactly what stress I had been under, learning to teach and dealing with new contracts that called all the part-time teachers at my work casual workers! They explained to me that my boys could come and see me near the end of my two weeks in hospital. My hubby had given me pictures of them which I had carried around. Occasionally other patients asked to see the pictures. Sometimes I would get paranoid again and be reluctant to show them.

When my boys did come they sat in a special visitors' room. They seemed remarkably OK and at last I knew that nothing bad had happened. I can't remember what we talked about but I think they had some toys or magazines to show me. My eldest had become very quiet when I was in hospital and I wish I could have seen him earlier but that would not have been a good idea, as he wouldn't have understood how I was behaving. They went home and I knew that they would be looked after.

I have some other snippets of memory from when I started to feel better in the ward. At one point I actually broke the fire alarm fitting at the end of the corridor. It was a way of trying to get out and escape. Not sure where I would have ended up if I had made it. We were let out usually once a day under close supervision to an activity area within a quad. I'd explore the quad and walk round it very fast as a form of exercise. It was also nice to sit in the sun. We would do quizzes, play table tennis and badminton. I particularly liked jewellery making and made bracelets for my various visitors including my auntie, mum-in-law and family friends. I also started colouring. Get some adult colouring books, they are great!

Back in the ward wasn't so bad, although I had figured out all the windows had cages for good reason. One day when I was lying on a mattress in the mattress room (not sure why), I heard some commotion outside. It was the police; they were bringing someone to the hospital. I shouted down to them, 'Do you know my husband?' At least by that time I knew what job he actually did and that he wasn't a teacher.

Occasionally I would have returning feelings about the conspiracy theory. One day I looked out of the window and thought I saw all the cars moving around the hospital. I moved around the building and saw cars moving at each window. I almost convinced myself that the government was involved and I was being watched.

Before I left the ward I wrote down all the rooms as I thought it would help me try and explain my illness.

The rooms in Sapphire were; Calming, Side Room 1–4, Dining Room, Lounge, Seclusion, Staff Room, Laundry, Sluice Room (I think this is the one that I read as suicide room), Toilets 1–7, Staff Toilet, Nursing Office, Manager's Office, Ward, Store Rooms 1 and 2 , Nursing Office, Dormitory 1–3, Clinical Room, Linen Room, and CRHT Office (I later looked this up as Crisis Resolution and Home Treatment), Ward Review Room, Bathroom, Shower Room, Domestic Room, Handover and Family Room, Doctors' Room, and one out of order toilet. Just typing this out reminds me of early on, knocking on the doors and asking for people involved in my conspiracy theory. I think while you're in the ward, notes are being made on what you are doing so they could review your progress.

I remember before my release I went before some kind of panel, a bit like when you are allowed out on parole, and I answered some questions. Flashbacks of a similar meeting before I was better came back, when I was wearing a hospital gown and a bit of a wreck.

Once I had been in the ward a while I realised the desk was where people seemed to meet before going down for activities. It was also where you had phone calls from the outside. I had quite regular phone calls from my sister. She had a one-year-old and lived in Birmingham with a full-time job so it wasn't easy for her to get down. I remember being really happy to talk to her. Can't remember what we talked about but I guess that doesn't matter.

Having showers and borrowing some hair-removal cream for my legs (for good reason we weren't allowed razors) also made me feel better. I guess when you are away with the fairies you forget about everyday tasks like hygiene and looking after your appearance. The shower rooms were pretty big and I remember singing out my problems in the shower. My key worker would knock to check where I was. Not sure if she heard my ramblings.

One time I was looking at the leaflets on the wall and leant against the wall singing, 'It's all about the money, money, money.' I think this related to losing out on my redundancy pay-out and the possibility of losing out on my golden hello (a reward payment for newly qualified science teachers) which I was working so hard towards. Or it may have been that the government had reduced police pensions and not that of MPs! With a smile on her face, my key worker asked if I was alright. I think she realised it was all part of getting better.

I had also written out how I had misinterpreted words that people were saying around me (see the table).

Word I heard	Word they actually said
Kill	Call
Dead	Instead
Police	Release
Arrest	A rest

I also wrote that mirrors were weird. Maybe it's because I had a habit of talking into them and then thought later that they may be two-way, probably because I've watched quite a lot of films! Another note that I'd made in hospital said 'can't trust' – then the name of the company that I worked for. It was signed at the bottom. I think this says a lot about work-related stress and how dangerous it can become.

A few days before I left I remember lying in bed to just before breakfast ended at 9. I think I hadn't had a good lie-in for a long while and this hadn't helped much. One of the nurses explained that I would have to move to the dormitory. This made me a bit anxious but I was next to a couple of people I got on with, so that was fine. In fact I had always felt safe in Sapphire Ward.

One night they locked us in the lounge area for a while as a new patient was resisting her admission. We could hear her in the seclusion room area shouting out and being restrained. When I saw her the next day she was a big lady. In the corridor she apologised for how she had been. I remember saying to her, 'Don't worry.' I could imagine her stress as she was held in the seclusion room wanting to get home. The seclusion room was basically a room with a blue mattress with an interconnecting room. I had explored there once and tried lying on the mattress, rocking as if to see if I had gone fully mad. I concluded in the end that I had been treated in time.

One of the ladies on the ward had been there a long time. She was very vocal but harmless enough and liked to dress up if there was an opportunity. Ironically she was fond of a fairy stick.

Other people I had met had evidence of self-harming on their arms. One girl with these marks had run away on our way back from activities. A nurse had managed to chase her and bring her back. I had learned that there was such a range of mental health issues and some people didn't get to go home as quickly as I had.

I don't remember when I was released but I remember packing and saying goodbye. As I walked out of the hospital with my husband it was surreal. We walked past everyone in their own individual worlds and past the coffee shop with people chatting and catching up. He drove me back in my car and it was good to get home, and I knew I'd have to keep an eye on my mental health from then on.

Chapter 5
Relapse

Well, after being released from hospital I had the summer to get it together. I bravely went to work in September but only managed a couple of weeks. I remember taking a lesson and thinking, 'Why am I doing this? I don't want to be here, what if I get ill again in front of the students?' So I phoned up the next day to say I wasn't going in. Luckily my parents were staying with me and I went to the doctors with my mum.

The doctor asked me a few questions and one was about had I thought about suicide. I had replied that I couldn't as I had two boys to think of and that was keeping me going. Luckily I still had logical thought which I know can go if you're really ill. She arranged for me to be signed off and I received counselling for six weeks.

I was told by the doctor to go out and enjoy doing things on my time off but I found even going out I couldn't relax or be happy. Mum and Dad were looking for a house nearer to us so we went to a few houses to look at them which helped. It took my mind off things and we'd discuss if the garage was big enough for all their vehicles etc. Shopping always helped but you can't do that all the time. Exercise didn't seem to help or maybe I wasn't doing it right or pushing myself enough.

The counselling I had been prescribed was useful. It got me to ask questions and come up with possible strategies about work, for example how to lighten my workload. I was still feeling depressed about not being able to cope. After my sign-off period I asked to go to zero hours; this was one advantage of my new contract. My head of department and vice-principal were understanding and later on let me go back on reduced hours. Returning to work was alright and it was nice to see everyone again. Although the planning for teaching lessons never really stops, and evenings and weekends can be swallowed up. The whole contract thing had blown over; it was now inspection time.

It was clear that inspection was everything and luckily as an NQT I would be spared a further inspection (the one previously had judged me just satisfactory as I had frozen in panic). But the trigger for my relapse was being observed by my vice-principal. The lesson had gone well and I was awarded a good which meant I had passed my NQT. However, it had taken its toll.

A few days later I had started to feel ill again in a lesson. The problem was that I had not prepared the lesson as there had been a misunderstanding about a school trip. So I went through some marked work with the students but then ran out of things to do with them. The head of the course, who was a very confident person, came in and I thought the conspiracy theory had started again. I thought it was all a set up and had to sit down and apologise to the students.

The lesson seemed to go on forever and I felt giddy. After the lesson I went to the staffroom and sat between my close friends, I was in shut-down mode and realised that I couldn't drive home. They sat with me and comforted me. I then went down to the office and rang my husband. Thank God he was in and he came to rescue me. I stayed in the office with the receptionist looking out for me.

I remember looking out of the window thinking that snipers were out there and that I should keep out of sight. It took a while for my hubby to arrive and one of my friends had come down to check on me. For a moment I didn't trust her and she could sense this. She said she would take me to her car and take me home but I kept thinking she was part of it so I panicked once we got to the door and walked back to the office. When my husband arrived I all but ran to the car and was so relieved. He drove me to the Beacon to get more medication. I don't remember consciously coming off them but we had no more at home.

I phoned the Beacon on the way and when they asked for my personal details I didn't give them any more than my name as I didn't trust giving personal details on the phone. Funny when you look back on it I guess. The mental health worker asked me some questions and I said what had happened at work which probably didn't make much sense. He got us a prescription and we went to Tesco for food and tablets. I remember even being paranoid about the food and whether it had been poisoned. I was checking the seals and everything.

We got home and I had a tablet and went to bed. Mum and Dad visited as we had phoned them from the Beacon. The next day I stayed off work and we went to a nearby seaside town for a coffee. I felt guilty again that I had the day off and wasn't visibly ill. I had gotten ill again really quickly but I seemed to be recovering quickly too.

Chapter 6
Medication

It was now August 2016 and I was told at my mental health review to record how I was feeling as I had decided to try and come off my olanzapine tablets. A GP had told me about six months before this that it was easy to come off them. I had asked myself at the time, how did he know?

About a week and a half later (less than three weeks after my last tablet) I had relented and taken a tablet. I wasn't sleeping well and the anxiety had become too much and I couldn't cope with the simplest of tasks. The thought of going back to work after the holiday was too much and I was waking up in a panic after some realistic dreams that were weird to say the least. One of my dreams involved my parents' boat and having to come back from a trip out due to the waves becoming really big. Once the boat was safely on the shore it shrank and I woke up. Other dreams involved weird multistorey parking or journeys on a conveyor belt.

I had reached a point where my anxiety was controlling me. The anxiety had stopped me going out apart from out into town by foot. I would worry about silly things such as scratches or damage on things around the house. I went for a walk to think about taking a tablet. When I got back I took one and the relief was almost instant. The effects were quite strong and I slurred my words. Luckily I didn't have to drive that day.

Once I had decided to take my tablets again I saw a couple of good friends and just talking things through with them helped. I was still turning to alcohol a fair bit to try and calm my nerves all the while I knew this wasn't the answer.

For now I would continue on my tablets as they were keeping my anxiety levels low enough to function.

People had started to notice my hand shake quite a bit so I returned to the doctor. He prescribed more tablets for anxiety and they seemed to be helping with this. Meanwhile I wasn't having much luck with my claim against my employer for everything my family and I had gone through. Still, it gave me focus.

There isn't much awareness of how mental health claims are handled and quite frankly one solicitor had been ignorant and dismissive about my 'date of knowledge' (for which there is leeway for in mental health matters). I had done quite a lot of research into mental health injury and thanks to the Yapp case, you have to prove that your employer a) could have foreseen how ill you would get and b) fail to take steps to prevent your illness. No one really saw how ill I was; although I was behaving in a rather strange way I had not emailed someone to say, 'Hey, I'm going to have a breakdown.' My solicitor, who I had found through the Law Society, was not only in touch with mental health he also cared about what was right.

Unfortunately after an hour on the phone and looking at the evidence I had, we decided it was a borderline case and to not pursue it any further. This was probably a good thing as visions of a courtroom made me anxious and I had already had minor signs of psychosis again just going through what had happened. I had looked at an unopened bottle of Coke in my fridge and because it wasn't that full I had a feeling it had been tampered with. Also, I had a thought for a few seconds that the house had been bugged and they could hear us discussing the case.

Chapter 7
So why did I have this breakdown?

Why should I ask this question? It just happened, right? After coming off my tablets in 2016 I got angry when I realised I had to go back on them and five years had not been enough to recover. Olanzapine dampens your emotions and I never really got angry about it all until then. Calming down, back on the tablets, I worked on finishing this account as it was therapeutic.

Well I am now certain in my own mind that it was due to the new contracts that were brought in at work and the lack of sleep due to my worry about these. They had been introduced at the end of term after pressure with lesson planning and looming inspections. They had been given out to us during an after school session. In fact they weren't even given out they were just left on the side for us. The part-time contract was particularly derogatory and incorrect. I had checked on a website and we were entitled to more than the contracts implied. Why hadn't someone checked before they were issued?

A group of us had discussed them the next day and we had even been to see the principal to voice our concerns. I remember being angry and on a mission as I did not want to lose the great atmosphere we had at work in the staffroom and between the teachers. After all, this is what kept me going at work.

I looked at the emails that were flying around at the time, although I did not have access to my work emails we had set up a mailing list with my private email and others so I have access to these. Just looking at them now is enough to show that the whole thing had been stressful in addition to training to teach and writing a course.

One of my friends at the school gate had asked if I was alright when I picked up my boys one day. I had said that we were just so worried about the contracts at work. She nodded in understanding but I guess she didn't know how ill I was getting. Otherwise she would have taken me out for retail therapy, believe me. She had taken me out before. I had tried a dress on, only I had thought it was a skirt. It was one of those new types of dresses that you just pull up. She had said, 'This is long overdue!'

Below are a few of my emails that I sent just before my breakdown:

It all started off as the staff group helping each other out.

I love working there too, but only if the staff/people don't change too much. They'll just get a load of teachers from Cambridge in if we walk out.

Hang on in there until we find out more. Keep all your pay slips as evidence that you are an employee. You've worked there more than I have, and you and Marie do a lot for the college.

This one shows when my paranoia began to set in.

I keep having sleepless nights and possibly rightly so. After the posts yesterday I feel we need to be very careful as fat salaries may be at stake which can make people stoop very low. I thought what if they infiltrated the group. They could even set up an email account with someone else's name. If they get hold of our emails they could try to break the group apart by sending messages to us.

This one shows the development of the conspiracy theory.

You're honest and you say it how you see it, even if it may upset (someone high up). Somebody out there isn't and I think it will come out soon.

All the best. I'm glad I'm not at work next term. Keep in touch.

This one was sent either on the day I went into hospital or the day before just to my head of department. I've learned to stay off my email more after all this. It can be a real battle ground.

I've finally figured it out after a few nights without much sleep. I will keep quiet as this needs sorting. You were very strong and now need the title Dr Inspector…

All the best and good luck.

We may need to all go off directory enquiries although it will be too late for some so they will need reassurance.

So, it was quite ironic that this email group set up to help may have contributed to my illness as things weren't adequately sorted before the holidays. I had tried to be the hero and it hadn't worked.

Chapter 8
Spotting the signs

Before I became ill the first time, I would go quiet, particularly at meal times. I would go off into my own world of anxiety. I couldn't even relax watching films. I had been drinking lots of Coke and the caffeine probably didn't help. I had stopped eating breakfast as it made me gag. I also had a particular mannerism where I would rub the left of my forehead. Mum and Dad are convinced I had a virus near the time which didn't help. I would also say, 'Ohhhhh!' In a particular way that my husband has learned to recognise. But the most important thing now is that I can tell when I'm getting ill and do something about it. Knowing when I'm manic is also a good thing.

One of my friends said I had been manic in the week before my 'psychotic episode'. I had bought a new dress for the graduation and was quite animated for the trash fashion show. One day before this someone had been run over outside the college. I had seen her with her head against the kerb being looked after by a passer-by. I directed the ambulance to her but could not face getting any closer so I went up to the staffroom and had to get a cup of tea. I did not calm down for a while and kept going over what happened.

When I left, the ambulance was still there in the road and the road was closed off. It was weird that I felt a darkness over me as I walked by. I found out later that she had survived and had run out from the bushes into the road in her nightwear. She had been suffering from poor mental health. Soon I would understand what this meant.

Later I found out that Sapphire Ward had been changed to ambulatory care (another needed resource) and mental health patients had to go further to get help. I hope some influential people read my account and understand how I was kept safe for two weeks.

Here's a poem I wrote before I left.

'On the ward'

I was scared!
I was tired!
I was angry!
But I didn't know why

I started to feel better
As I started to see where I was,
My kids were OK
But I needed to see them

I had lots of visitors and people around were nice,
When my boys came,
They were strong and happy so I was too.

I want to go home to sort out my life
But I need to rest
That's the test… Sapphire Ward.

PART 2
...and beyond

Chapter 1
How did I get here?

In a way working at the school I was now at was similar to my time spent in Sapphire Ward in hospital: the erratic behaviour of the students, the fire alarms and the wandering in corridors. The patients were more courteous though and we would line up for our tablets at night and our blood pressure check in the morning. So how did I end up in this 'hard school' as described by a supply teacher with more than twenty-five years' experience?

Well, it had all started when redundancies came in at work where I was an analytical chemist. I had experience of working with young people when I had done volunteer work. So I thought teaching; surely that would be rewarding. I got a place on a PGCE course and started out at a local Catholic school. The staff were really nice and I enjoyed my first placement. It was a bit of a shock when I started my second placement. The staff weren't as friendly and the pressure of the selective school was apparent. I had made a rocky start at the second school probably not helped by my ignorance of what such a school would be like. Also, I was late on my first day due to not being able to drop my children off until 8, and roadworks on the way in. I remember thinking it would be easier there.

How wrong could I be? I failed my first visit by my tutor and it all looked as if it was over. But I managed to carry on and seemed to get respect for that. A lot of people were off sick and I would step in where I could. I remember my mentor being physically sick outside the form room once so I took over. I wasn't observed as much as I should have been, but my mentor's daughter would be in the lesson occasionally and she must have given positive feedback about the role plays I was doing for active learning.

I think it was during this placement that I started to neglect my mental health needs. At the end of it all when I managed to pass I remember rewarding myself with a bath and a beer! One thing I did know was that I'd never go back to that school.

At the time I was learning to teach there were over thirty TDA standards to be met for qualified teacher status. The ones I found most difficult were:

1: Have high expectations of children and young people including a commitment to ensuring that they can achieve their full educational potential and to establishing fair, respectful, trusting, supportive and constructive relationships with them.

38: Use a range of behaviour management techniques and strategies, adapting them as necessary to promote the self-control and independence of learners.

I found these two clashed somewhat. Some classes only responded to a good shouting at or numerous detentions being given out. Shouting at a whole class wasn't necessarily fair as some students were not to blame. Giving detentions sometimes did not help with trust. I recently gave a detention out to someone in a class for constant mobile phone use. She got quite aggressive about this and swore at me using the F word. 'I'm not going to detention,' she shouted. 'I have a mum to go home to.' Then turning to her friend, 'I hate her, she's not even a proper teacher.' After all, she wasn't to know I was actually a fully qualified teacher, with four years' experience, and I had chosen to not be a teacher any more due to stress. I was now a science tutor. Some students had become 'resistant' to learning and it would take a long time and adequate resources for independent learning to develop.

One of my colleagues likened meeting these standards to jumping through hoops. We were also taught to be reflective, this was all well and good but inevitably ended up with the trainee teacher blaming everything on themselves, which is never good for mental health. Some phrases used when writing these reflections were: I should have… I could have… and I would have…. . The trainee teacher would then explain why doing what they had done was a mistake. After a while it became equivalent to beating yourself with a large stick.

After training it would be a year before I got a permanent job in teaching, though I did spend a few days in a pupil referral unit. I kind of fitted in there as I was patient and not too overpowering with the kids. Notably I managed to keep a runaway kid inside the unit. We did some coursework and then played table tennis. He had his issues, body odour being one of them, but I helped him as much as I could. These were kids that couldn't cope with main stream and it would be valuable experience for the future.

Whilst looking for a job I had to sign on at the local Job Centre and this was an experience in itself. The advisers were OK apart from the one at the end who said he didn't want to see me back there after paying for my Smart Board Course! There were teaching jobs coming up but I was adamant I wanted a job that I could handle, part-time would be best although I later learned there was no such thing as a part-time teacher. One thing I found strange about the Job Centre was that there were security guards there. There was no money handled so I think it was to protect the staff from abuse. Luckily I could go when the children were in school so I didn't have to take them. I had signed up with a couple of agencies and they would ring me with some unsuitable jobs from time to time such as a job which was miles away at Folkestone Academy.

The interview wasn't too disastrous but my heart wasn't in it as it was too far away; yeah, like that would fit in with the school run! I stayed for lunch at the interview and managed to catch up with someone who used to be my mentor. After lunch I went home as I thought that was the end. The agency was not best pleased as they said I could have got the job. Never mind if I wanted it or not!

I had got my teaching position in 2010. A year later I had my nervous breakdown. After which one of my friends had jokingly said it was because I lived with my husband, she told him as much. She said, 'No, really it's because she lives with you!' She knew him well as she worked with him!

Mental health of women is said to be worse when married but I didn't blame my husband, in fact he had always supported me. OK little criticisms about how I loaded the dishwasher didn't help, but he had his particular way of doing things and he knew if I did things slapdash this was an indicator of my health.

I also had other issues; only the other day I caught myself checking the glass pane on the kitchen door for a scratch as I had accidently bashed it with my engagement ring. I even cleaned it up, paranoid that I had caused damage. A doctor had recently annoyed me. I had expressed my concern over my son becoming anxious and had reminded her of my problems. She had rather matter-of-factly replied that, 'I should be careful how I acted around my children as they would learn this behaviour.' It was made worse that she said this in front of my son so he would remind me of this. But if my sons saw me doing anything strange it was probably good that they pointed it out.

A while after my breakdown I saw a change of job, a role as a teaching assistant, advertised closer to home. So I went for it. The interview was pretty strenuous and when they phoned up to say I'd got it, I couldn't believe it. It was great news; I had gone for so many jobs. I could leave planning lessons in the past and it was near home so I would be nearby for my kids. So I started in the September. I remember on my first day a fight had broken out and the student involved walked out of the sports hall. I followed him and he punched the bin hurting his hand. Luckily a more experienced PE teacher dealt with the student, it was all a bit of a shock.

I found my time in the family unit particularly rewarding as this was mostly 1:1. I found myself getting drawn to science again and would set up experiments for them to do in the family unit. The students appreciated it, one of them would talk quite a bit about his knowledge of science and I wished I had more equipment. About a year in I decided to go for the science tutor role (thirty-three hours a week). The role as it was then was to help in lessons, take small groups for intervention, help with marking, create spreadsheets and to supervise coursework catch ups. It was a scary step as I knew that the workload may make me ill again if I wasn't careful.

Chapter 2
Telling my employers

That was a hard conversation. After the six week break I decided to tell the HR manager that I was on anxiety tablets. She was understanding and explained that someone she knew had similar problems. It was a while before I told my head of department. She had come into my room and had sat down to do her work. I thought it's now or never; we were always so busy. The topic came up as we were talking about stress. I think I said, 'I've had problems in the past and I'm now on tablets for it.' She said, 'Oh no, make sure you take care.' She started to check if it was anything in particular. I replied, 'No, it's not this job it was my last job.' Which I have to say wasn't entirely the truth. After all, we were all under a lot of stress in the school. I'd just learned to deal with it. Not necessarily to not care about the workload but to manage to deal with it.

The term had started in a surreal way; strict new rules on uniform had been introduced by the new Head. So strict in fact, that the media had become involved. Media vans were waiting outside in the morning and I had to walk past them, all the while conscious that I may get asked something or my clothing may be scrutinised. Some parents and students were grouping up outside talking to the media. It made me feel nervy and I would walk in as quickly as possible. I was aware of a slight darkening around me as I walked in, similar to what I had felt outside my old work when the woman had got hit by the car. Friends would text to see how I was coping with all the commotion.

We had a false impression that behaviour was improving in the school straight away, as a lot of students had not been let in. That would soon change.

I had seen a friend when collecting my medication tablets we had talked about work making us ill. The man giving me the tablets said, 'Do you get these free?' I looked through the list of reasons to get free medication and didn't seem to meet any. I quite openly said it was for mental health and he went out back to check. Unfortunately it didn't count which seemed a little unfair particularly as it had all been caused by work-related stress and overload. It came to £16.80. I knew that this may be every couple of months for the rest of my life. I reminded myself that the tablets were keeping me well and that my husband had said I was more like my old self since taking the day-time ones. I was starting to smile more and joke more at home.

I still had underlying worries; didn't everyone have these? Sometimes these came out as dreams. I had woken up from another really vivid dream but at least it was half term so I didn't have to face work. The dream had involved our shared driveway out front. Apparently the neighbours, who were away, had let their friends set-up camp there. I remember trying to reason with their friends as they parked their vehicles in our way and moved their caravans in, it ended up with me hurling abuse at them. Some of them had invaded our house and I had managed to get them out – apart from two girls who seemed harmless enough. Maybe it was time to go on stronger tablets but I didn't really want to.

Students at school also seemed to suffer similar problems. I was walking back to my room in school when a student came up to me explaining that someone needed a teacher as she was having a panic attack. I walked with her up some stairs to the side of a building. The girl was lying down and in a bad way. She was pulling at her tie and had managed to undo it a little. She was coughing and had excess saliva. I managed to get her up with another student's help and we walked slowly, supporting her when she became wobbly. We got to one of the labs and sat her down for a while, reassuring her and asking her questions. I managed to untie her tie and my boss stayed with her before taking her to student services.

Staff were caring at our school, you had to be. One day I heard a conversation outside my room between patrol and a Year 11 student. It was about a seating plan change that the student didn't agree with. It went something like this:

'You need to just go in there and sit where you are asked.'

'She's treating me like a dickhead in front of my friends.'

'I just want to sit where I usually do.'

'I'm missing out on learning.'

'Yes, that's why you need to get in there and get on with your test, or you can sit in here (meaning my room).'

'I'm struggling with life, I hate her, you know how stubborn I am!'

Eventually the negotiating skills of the teacher and patrol won. The student was at least honest about her feelings but it shows what disruption can be caused by one student against one simple rule. In a full class of thirty this could become a big issue.

All half term I had experienced nightmares about work but at least my anxiety had fallen thanks mainly to a break away in Earnley where life was more relaxed. The most vivid dream that I had had was of my head of department being observed by the Head teacher. The lesson was going OK and at least the students were in their seats and in the correct uniform.

The Head walked in late and seemed not to care about

what was going on. He started writing random stuff on the white board all the while being abusive to my head of department. I was glad to wake up but I knew that work was affecting my health again and I would need coping mechanisms.

Chapter 3
My coping mechanisms

Spending time with my kids definitely helped and my week away with my sister and our kids had relaxed me completely. I would have some alcohol in the evening although you are not supposed to on my tablets mainly because it makes you drowsy, but I found it helped me to reboot. I knew I was reliant on alcohol but what with working full-time and my husband working long hours, it helped. After all, I only had at the max two beers in the evening.

Time with one of my best friends every Saturday morning was also a coping mechanism. I would have a coffee and we'd have a good chat and a laugh, tears only came once, when her dad was seriously ill. We'd go out for a walk with her dog and the kids. Even then I would become anxious. One of her twins asked why my hands were wobbly and I explained I was taking tablets for it.

We would walk the dog to some sunken gardens near her house. The kids would run off into the bushes that surrounded the garden. When they disappeared I would have thoughts that they may have been abducted. I knew these were just thoughts but they would pop up and I would try to control them. We would call out and they'd shout back or poke their heads up. One day we went down there and the bushes had been cut back so there were fewer places to hide. This made me feel better but some of the fun had gone for the kids, like modern life I guess. It was always good to see my friend; we'd each discuss our problems and comment on the week's events. Even watching cooking programmes with her was good. I'm not even interested in cooking!

One Saturday I was driving back from seeing her. There was a right turn near the seafront and it was close to another T-junction. I looked both ways and saw someone was coming, after they turned I looked again and decided to move out. I saw someone had just turned into the road. I made the snap decision to continue to come out as I was committed. As I turned I could see that they had slowed down a little but they had changed direction. Surely they weren't going to ram us? My son in the back noticed too. I moved out of the way as quickly as possible. I knew it was important to get away from them so continued going looking back once to see they had stopped their car.

We were relieved to get home and I explained that some drivers did this to claim insurance money. I reached for an anxiety tablet and managed to calm myself.

My next big coping mechanism was to get home and check Facebook. It was an excellent way to keep in touch with people that I hadn't seen for ages. I recently put a post on it about my dreams.

'If you work in a highly stressful environment your dreams may be outrageous and vivid.' Oh dear, I'd been having them for months now.

There were quite a few comments on this:

'I have weird dreams all the time.'

'I hope you're looking after yourself, Mrs?? Xx.'

'I must have been stressed all my life then, my dreams are just weird xx.' (This friend had also suffered night walking, one night attacking a clothes airer in her room!)

'Join the club!'

'I'm too tired from teaching and marking to have dreams. Also not in bed long enough! X'

I replied: 'OK I'm quite normal then.'

I'd also put a few comments on mental health on Facebook.

One comment was:

'Managed to get as far as the local country house today. Anxiety sucks but the more I get out and do things the easier it gets. Boys liked maze and bloke dressed up in chicken costume with water pistol was funny.'

'Anxiety?' was a reply from someone I had worked closely with for over a year. I think I must have hidden my symptoms well then, which is not always a good thing.

What with all the people dressed up as clowns lately we were lucky it was just a chicken costume. At school someone had poked their head into my room wearing some sort of Halloween mask. It hadn't scared me as I'd learned to expect the unexpected at work.

I had also put a post on Facebook about how the media had been more concerned about what the Duchess of Cambridge was wearing on the Mental Health Awareness Day, not on what work she had been doing towards it!

Writing about my experiences had recently become a coping mechanism. I am sitting here now with a pile of ironing in the other room but I choose to leave that for the moment as this is more therapeutic. At my yearly review a doctor had advised me to write a diary about my feelings, in fairness I had already started writing so that my children had some sort of answer if they wanted to know. The doctor was concerned that I would need a way of not getting to crisis point again. She had been the one who advised me to tell someone at work about my anxiety. I knew she was right and to be honest I didn't mind talking about it, I just didn't want it to be seen as an excuse. After all one of our new aims at school was 'there are no excuses'.

Chapter 4
In front of the chaos

Two people had left that September due to stress. One had just come in one day seen how the students were and how much work had to be done before going off ill. The other, a student teacher, had at least made two weeks before deciding it wasn't for him. However, all this had impacted on those of us that remained. I was constantly being called on to cover lessons despite having my own work to do.

One particular cover lesson I will always remember is described here. It was in S1, a room downstairs, and the class had a lot of English Additional Language needs. Despite this there was no one in to support me. The lesson started off quite tamely but an atmosphere started to build in the room. Two students seemed particularly interactive. One moved over to the other and I should have made him sit back in his seat straight away. A few of the class said, 'It's OK; they are best friends.'

Time seemed to stay still and then the class started chanting. I quickly moved over to the two students who were now standing up and moving to the back of the classroom. There was a scuffle and I shouted out to one of the students to go and get the head of department. The noise level got pretty high and I moved between the students, and my pass was pulled off in the commotion.

My head of department came in and shepherded one of the students into another room. The buzzer went and the students left leaving me to deal with my emotions and to thank the students who had held back those that were fighting.

I had to go and check if any students had turned up to my next lesson although they weren't expected. My head of department saw me when I returned to my room and asked me if I was OK. I managed a reply but was still a bit shaken. I wrote up the incident and asked for alarm buttons but to no avail. We had phones but a complicated login procedure was needed before you got anywhere.

I have also survived two lessons in front of the most notorious Year 8 class. The class came in and took ages to settle, this of course was not helped by me not knowing their names, although I soon picked up on the names of the most troublesome ones. At one point I was just moving my hands up and down and saying 'calm down'. I must have resembled the Scousers who said 'calm down, calm down' on *The Harry Enfield Show*. The new teacher with me was also overwhelmed and concentrated on small groups and stopping students from going into the next classroom.

Eventually the noise level dropped, I had drawn a spider diagram on the board and it was to do with the three states of matter. I had been told on my PGCE to write down any input from the students so when one of the students shouted out 'fart' for gas I was obliged to write it down. Some of the students found this funny and seemed to settle down and get on with some of the work. I had to praise the class quite a lot and even said the noise level was good which wasn't entirely true. Somehow the teacher and I survived until the buzzer and we then had to tidy up the mess in the classroom, all the while reflecting on our experience. I even said it was better than I expected!

The next lesson with this class was worse in a way because no one seemed to settle. The warning systems set up seemed to fail. You would get a student to pay attention and then another would start. One child had spat on another's blazer so I got my tissues out, eventually senior management came and they got the class to practise sitting quietly. The individual students on their own were not too challenging but as a group it was a hard task to control. The new teacher who had this group added to her timetable was in tears after a lesson with them. I could totally relate to how difficult it could be moving schools and starting out, and tried to comfort her as much as possible.

This is a quote from my PGCE report at my second school placement:

'This was an additional visit approved by the subject leader, because of the award of a Grade 4 (fail) for professional skills on the first visit. At the time of the last visit, Samantha was lacking confidence and was not demonstrating the level of competence in her teaching skills that she showed in her Level 2 placement… Today's visit confirmed that she has made steady progress.'

Thank goodness I had a tutor who didn't give up on me. I too had been in the staffroom in tears at one point.

My confidence did go up and down and I did try to appear confident even if I wanted the floor to swallow me up. Our drama teacher had commented on the Year 8s. He had had both of the hardest Year 8 classes in the hall for a session. He said it was the worst experience of his life, and he had nearly died twice in his life! He was a very confident teacher and I wish I could have been more like that.

I had become a reluctant teacher that was now a science tutor and who was coping day by day. Don't get me wrong, there were some good bits to teaching, the occasional 'Thank you, Miss', 'I get science now' and a student going 'Wow' when they look down a microscope at the holes in a leaf. I recently found a thank you card from a Year 9 class who I had taught about food chains using cuddly toys. Some of the comments were heart-warming. 'Thanks for teaching us', 'Will miss you', 'I love science well bad'. I will always keep that card; to me it helps remind me why I do my job. Maybe most of my failings were in my head and I was doing a good job.

I found that exam answers were sometimes a source of amusement and this helped when marking piles of them. There was a question describing the differences between snails and slugs. Most of the students referred to the snail having a home and the slug not. One pointed out that this was sad for the slug. Sweet but not entirely scientifically correct.

Chapter 5
Similarities to Sapphire Ward

It was around this time that five fire alarms were set off in one day. Luckily it wasn't a rainy day. Two had been set off before lunch. I had cleared my room and gone out to the tennis courts where we all assembled. I had stood where the other support staff were standing. We commented on who might have set them off. This would all be recorded on CCTV cameras scattered around the school and an email usually went out after the culprit had been found. The third time it was just before lunch so students and staff were worried about getting time for lunch, in the event extra time was given. We thought that was it but we were again disturbed after lunch. I remember walking out saying, 'This about sums it up, doesn't it?' I was referring to behaviour. We were just being let in when the alarm sounded again. I recall looking out of the window seeing the confused students on the grass area. It reminded me of the time I looked out of the Sapphire Ward window to see all the cars moving round. Only this time I knew the situation was real. Eventually we could continue with lessons and luckily there seemed to be no repeat of this day.

Another gentle reminder of my stay in hospital was some students singing as they walked past my room. The heating had been turned on. 'It's getting hot in here, let's take off all our clothes' I smiled to myself as I had a brief flashback of my false or true memory of walking down the corridor in Sapphire Ward half dressed. It was good to be reminded of being ill as it served to remind me to take care.

A good indicator of if I was well or not, was to monitor my mild OCD. For instance, I would regularly check my wallet to see if my cash card was in it. I'd lie in bed suddenly remember then go down to look in my wallet. I also had to check the house quite a lot before I went out. Was the back door locked? Was the iron unplugged (yes probably as I was too distracted to iron lately!)? Were the gas burners off? Had I shut the front door properly? Every morning as I arrived at work I would check the car door light was off, the interior light, the actual lights, the handbrake was on and the doors locked. An ex-student would see me sometimes, she must have thought I was mad.

It was weird how I could be OCD about some things but slapdash about others. I was sticking in some worksheets that my class had done (mainly because I didn't have enough glue sticks for them to do this in class). I had rather slapdashedly stuck some of them in with the edge sticking over the page. On handing them out one rather vocal student shouted out, 'Whose stuck this in my book? It's over the edge. I have OCD, I'm going to tear it out and write it out again!' Another girl copied this and tore it out. I explained that I'd been trying to help. I had no idea if they really had mild OCD or not (severe would have been recorded on the school system) but was willing to give them the benefit of the doubt, after all I had the rest of the class to teach.

Chapter 6
Restraint and retreat

Also, like Sapphire Ward and A and E, physical restraint was sometimes needed. A new leaflet had appeared on the table in the staffroom and it referred to physical restraint. I had seen how more experienced staff handled this. The first time I witnessed it was in the family unit and a regular student was walked in with a teacher on either side of him. They got him into one of the side rooms. I was working with another student at the time but I could hear some of what they were saying. They were reassuring him and saying at some point they would need a written statement from him. Their voices were calm and they were clearly skilled at this sort of thing. At no point did the student try to leave or harm himself any further.

Another time was when a student was threatening a teacher in the next room to mine. The head of maths was in there with a cover teacher helping with the situation. The student decided to walk into my room and started to talk to me as I was working on spreadsheets. They asked, 'Are you always in this room? What do you do all day?' I attempted to answer their questions not realising at first what the situation was and the student tried to get back in the classroom, the head of maths was now standing in front of the door with the other teacher. Patrol had also been called. They physically had to hold the door, all the while the student was trying to get past and push against them. I got up and moved over with the patrol lady.

We now had the student's bag and said, 'Come on; this way with your stuff.' But the student was not obliging; in the end they ran off round the building only to be prevented from being let into the classroom on the other side.

Another incident this time just requiring physical separation and again the help of a student was a Year 7 fight. I had come across it in the corridor; a Year 7 student was clearly upset. 'You're ruining my life,' he shouted at another student, his face red with anger. I followed him trying to get him to stop. A group of them went out into the playground where the argument continued and was soon going to get physical. A large number of people moved over keen to get in on the action. I looked around to see if there were any teachers for a moment I didn't see any and tried to get the students to move away. Another teacher came and helped to move people away. The student who was upset started to move back into the building as the head of maths came out and the boy was skilfully led into another room with another student's help. At this point I saw a colleague and told her what had happened. She had jokily replied, 'They're only Year 7s; can't take you anywhere,' implying that it could have been worse. I smiled; indeed Year 7s were less intimidating then say a tall Year 11 student.

Another example of when physical contact was required was in a Year 8 lesson, where a student decided five minutes before the end of the lesson to surf a stool which had fallen to the floor. Verbal instruction had failed to get him off; the noise level in the class did not help. Seeing imminent injury one of my colleagues quickly lifted him safely to the floor.

The staffroom was a place of retreat although even then some students would try to communicate through the window. One colleague was known for his outlandish comments in the staffroom and we all loved him for that, it was needed to keep the rest of us going. I noticed that the Union posters had been taken off the wall. I tried to keep all paranoid thoughts about why this was done out of my head, as I didn't want to go down the road that the appalling handling of my contracts at my old place of work had taken me. I was older and wiser now.

We were off to Thailand soon to see my father-in-law and all the family. I was looking forward to it as it meant a break from all the stresses of Christmas. But in another way I was in denial that we were going. There were an exponential number of things that could go wrong. The nurse who had given us injections for the trip had been quite frank about diseases out there. What if…? But again I had to be rational; it had been years since my children had seen their grandpa and one hadn't even met his grandma. We had a world map in one of our rooms and they would regularly look at this to see places they could travel to.

Sometimes I couldn't even retreat into my daydreams as thoughts would often pop up, in a way it was better if I was busy so they didn't. I could recognise irrational thoughts when I was well. See the table on the next page for how I would try to combat them:

Irrational thought that would pop into my head	How I dealt with them
'They've not come back from their fishing trip yet; maybe there's a problem, and maybe one has fallen over the side!'	I'm standing right by the coastguard boat and it's not been called out. One of them would have radioed in or contacted me somehow.
'OK, but what if the boat has sunk?'	They've all got life jackets on. There is a small life raft and they have a hand-held radio. (At which point my negative voice in my head seemed to run out of more horrific ideas.)
'The boys are with Mum and Dad, they haven't sent a text for a while. Maybe something's happened to them?'	They are just having a good time, silly. They all have a phone in case they get split up or get taken ill.
'He's been out with his friend longer than expected. Maybe he's been hurt?'	One of them has their phone! You've got to let them go sooner or later.
'Did I put their packed lunch in their bags?'	They won't starve, they have money in their bags and surely their friends will sell them some food!
We are in the woods and don't know exactly where we are. Everywhere looks the same; we'll never get back to the car.	If we keep walking one way we will find a road or the car park; we could survive one night out here if we had to, we had some drinks and food. (Since this experience I invested in some orienteering equipment!)

Quite frankly the future scared me silly but I just had to 'be strong' and to learn I couldn't control everything. People I knew were generally really supportive. 'I don't want you having a melt-down or anything.' If said in the right tone made me smile.

Sometimes there would be a less than helpful comment such as, 'You need to get a grip.' I too had been guilty of such comments; years ago my friend had got depression. I had simply said, 'Why are you depressed?' as if she had no need to be. She had looked at me exasperated but I think I understand more now. For instance, I had learned that anxiety would sometimes stop you doing things and then you would get depressed about the situation.

Recently we had taken time out as the kids were at my parents' and sat down and watched *Side Effects*. There were quite a few comparisons to my experience of mental health even though it turns out she wasn't actually ill it was all a ploy. It had shown her by the desk in the ward similar to where I had received phone calls. It also showed her driving into a wall, a similar thing had very briefly crossed my mind during the hardest times. On a happier note the film starred Jude Law. I joked about my hubby looking like him. Once he had told his work colleagues that I had said he looked like a cross between Jude Law and Daniel Craig. They had said, 'Hang on a minute, doesn't your wife have mental health issues?' I was glad he had banter at work I knew this helped him cope with the stresses of being in the police.

It was good to spend some quality time with my husband and he had said this too. We had also been to see *The Woman in Black* at the theatre for my birthday treat. Oddly this had not made my nightmares any worse and I hadn't imagined the woman in black in the back of the car on the way home, as I had done after watching the film. It had made me more determined to write my story and get it told, as this was what the first couple of scenes were about in the play.

Chapter 7
Looking into the past

It was at this stage that I started to look into my past further to see if there were any further reasons for my anxiety and paranoia. Yes there were instances; for example a group of school friends went up to Edinburgh for a hen weekend. The weekend was going well; we had done a bus tour, seen the dungeons with some scary actors adding dramatic tension, and frequented a few nightclubs.

I have this squint that wasn't totally corrected by an operation when I was five. So when I became tired my left eye wandered. On one of the last nights we went to a comedy night. We were sat near the front. The first act was OK and then for the second act he came on and immediately joked about my eyes wandering. I should have thrown some old cabbage at him but just sat there and took it.

I had been a bit paranoid when I was about eight, about something different. We had all gone out with the family to a pub garden. My nan had fallen over trying to get out of those pub benches. Luckily she hadn't hurt herself. On the way back the others were giggling and I thought it was all about me so I was in tears. Everyone explained they weren't laughing at me, but I was still upset.

It's weird what you remember sometimes. My sister and I had endured some bullying at our comprehensive school. I remember a few students had turned on us because I had said my best friend was my sister not another girl. So a couple who used to be close friends would sit behind us in geography all the while talking about us. They would try to cause problems between me and my sister by saying embarrassing things that we had each shared with them about our sister. Luckily my sister and I held strong together and moved onto another school in the end.

As for anxiety, I've always been a nervous person. I wasn't happy unless I was worrying about something. One incident again occurred when I was about eight or a little older. We had gone down to a beach near Chalkwell with some family friends. My sister and I and our two friends were playing on the breakwater. We were having a great time jumping off the posts and then climbing on again. The swell was pretty strong and I got in to trouble when I pushed myself too far off the breakwater. I was out of my depth and in a short while I realised I couldn't get back to the breakwater. I started to panic. I felt myself getting pulled under. I can still see it now, the sky becoming water as I went under for what seemed like six times. Each time I surfaced I waved my arms and I think I cried out but can't be sure.

Just when I thought I couldn't go under any more my friend called out and got me to climb on his back. He swam with me on his back until I was able to climb on the breakwater. Eventually I was about halfway along the breakwater and could walk up to the beach. My dad met me at the shoreline; they had been on the beach so didn't see the commotion straight away. I sat down on my towel shaking from my experience. People asked if I was alright but I remember being more embarrassed than afraid at this point.

Another incident involving water was when I went diving in a quarry in North Wales. The dive was going well and the visibility was great; we stopped at about ten metres and decided to try breathing with a spare regulator. I let go of my regulator and grabbed hold of the spare. I couldn't for the life of me get any air out of it. Again I started to panic and felt the urge to breathe; I even went to grab my instructor's regulator. She signalled me to use my existing regulator so we grabbed that and luckily it was working. She checked I was OK then we went to the shore.

Again, like my previous experience, we didn't discuss it afterwards and I'm not sure how scarred I was from it all but I did give up diving shortly after this.

Things had also been tough in later life when my son had been born premature and had become ill in hospital during his five-week stay there. More recently my husband had to be admitted to hospital for a serious infection. They had recovered but I, like many people, had lost people close to me and would in the future.

So I had had some reasons to be anxious and paranoid. I think when you are pushed to the limit for whatever circumstance (teaching and contracts in my case) your mental health is exhibited by the traits you are prone to. Recognising this has helped me understand my illness.

Chapter 8
Combating my feelings

I remember one senior manager admitting that standing in front of a class of Year 10s filled him with dread too. It was weird how now I didn't get nervous when asked to do short-notice cover, where I didn't really know the group, or have much to keep them entertained apart from a few instructions and book pages.

Just the other day I was asked to cover quite a difficult class. I looked at the attendance register on SIMS and cheered to myself that most of them were not in for whatever reason. I brushed up on what they were expected to do and dutifully went to the lesson five minutes early. They came in and I got the books out. 'Miss, we've already done this this morning!' I checked their books as you couldn't always believe them. They had done most of the work so I thought on my feet and moved them on a little.

Despite my best efforts only about half of the group did what they were asked. It was a constant battle. One student produced a football so I got him to put it back in his bag. Another student would not take her coat off as it was freezing. In fact it was cold as the remaining site team member who had known how to work the heating had been made redundant. I negotiated with her to put her phone away but to keep her coat on providing she also had her blazer on which she did have. Another student kept leaving and coming back, in the end I put 'quit' on the register for him.

Meanwhile others were working hard so they got house points. A student had sneaked in escaping from another lesson where she was allegedly being bullied by another student. A student had asked to go and get her asthma pump, so I had given her permission to get that, she then tried to go out again saying she hadn't got it. Another student had tried to escape via the fire escape so I had to deal with that. Two other students antagonized each other, the girl saying that he had been to the toilet in his pants and then swearing at him. I tackled this behaviour and she shouted, 'Why do you believe him and not me?' Erm... 'Because I've only seen your actions to him,' I replied. This all had to be logged as a serious behaviour after the lesson.

It was a Friday and instead of my bright and breezy feeling which I had briefly had in the morning I again felt like I had been run over by a bus! I said to my colleagues that I think I've put everything I can into the job feeling like this, and my colleagues joked about how much wine I would need tonight. I just couldn't fathom how teachers could deal with this kind of behaviour for up to six lessons a day and then plan in the evening for the next day. I was glad to help the teachers when I could and I felt appreciated. More help needed to be given and as far as I could see the government was only making things worse. The school had missed out on a 'build the schools for the future' promise and the building was quite frankly falling down. Over the day, food and wrappers would appear on the stairs and corridors. How was this supposed to inspire students? The number of support staff had been cut dramatically and resources were heavily limited. We weren't even able to photocopy worksheets for lessons and there was a freeze on ordering equipment. I had been to training on behavioural management and the main reason students don't behave is if they can't engage with the learning. I mean, come on, it's not rocket science; schools need more resources especially struggling ones! If students were helped earlier on, wouldn't there be less social problems in the future? I remember at my graduation a Dean had said that 'the price of education was high but the price of no education was higher'.

I had only really gone into a blind panic once or twice this term. Once was about the massive spreadsheet I had created for coursework. For a moment I thought I had saved over the most recent version with all the up to date classes. I had been noticing when this sort of thing happened I would find words hard to read on my laptop, I sometimes also got mild chest pains. I looked up symptoms of anxiety on the web and sure enough there they were. In a way I was relieved as maybe I could live with these short term problems. I'd be more vocal about my feelings and this would help. 'It's all getting a bit much,' I would say and people would listen.

The other time I had gone into a panic at work was when I nearly lost my laptop. I was doing another cover lesson and was writing some work on the white board. I turned round and my laptop had disappeared. My heart sank; the laptop was my main tool for everyday life, students were registered on it, behaviour was logged on it, presentations were shown on it, spreadsheets were on it, emails and documents. I could feel myself getting more and more worried. The class was looking for my reaction; no one was laughing. I said something like, 'You need to give me my laptop back. Who's got it?' and I started looking around the room. I started to examine everyone's faces to try and see who knew where it was continually asking, 'Where is it?'

Eventually, after what seemed like ages, a student got up and moved over to the fire escape. It had been hidden under a coat near the fire escape. I couldn't be sure who had taken it and went back to the front of the classroom. I decided it was just a prank and nothing too malicious. I was glad I kept my handbag on me at all times; if that was misplaced I wouldn't be able to get back home!

'You could write a book about this place,' I said to a colleague in the staffroom. 'No one would believe it!' she replied.

Having said that, things were slowly getting better; a new system had been set up so that students couldn't tear up their detention slips before they took them home. A text or email was sent straight to their homes, he-he. I even felt brave enough to visit the canteen at lunchtime for the first time since I started. The enticing power of sponge pudding and custard had won. It was well worth the trip.

I would go into work not knowing what I would face and sometimes feel like going home. In the end I must hold onto calm moments as people or situations can take these away. I had realised it took a special type of person to survive at our school and I had managed over two years there. Maybe I was this special kind of person, but what would be the cost?

PART 3

So I've trained as a science teacher, now it's time to look at the science of what happened and how it can help me. I've always enjoyed research. After I was ill someone at the Beacon had tried to explain it was due to a stress hormone and the effect on the brain. Maybe it's time I started to search for more answers. Here is what I've found.

The science behind it all

I've been struggling with names lately. Students would come into my room and I would look at their faces and try and remember their names – well there were quite a few Year 11s. I'd then say, 'What's your surname?' This would help me remember their first names. It wasn't for all students but I was struggling more lately probably as I had been feeling stressed. The stress hormone cortisol can play havoc with your memories. Furthermore, chronically elevated cortisol levels seem to impair memory [30]. It was quite stressful when specific students came in and their coursework needed to be found. Cortisol is released from the adrenal glands which are on top of the kidneys and transported in the blood, a trigger for its release is being anxious or stressed. I no longer coped with being nervous. Mum said, 'Everyone gets nervous.' But I knew it had made me ill in the past so I was keen to not feel that way wherever possible. However, 'Stress is unavoidable' [1], yes this was true even if I hibernated at home there were everyday worries about the kids and money for example.

'In addition there has been a long-standing association between raised or impaired regulation of cortisol levels and a number of psychiatric conditions such as anxiety and depression. However, the significance of this is not yet clearly understood.' [25] Why is it not clearly understood?

There have been various tests to see the effect of cortisol. One study was able to look at the data from cortisol levels, they looked at levels for healthy controls (people with no symptoms) and those at risk from psychosis including some mental health patients. The study [3] was heavy going for me even with a degree and a PGCE. Levels of cortisol can be tested using blood or saliva samples. This review seemed to show a link between anxiety and cortisol levels but was less conclusive for psychosis. I would need to investigate further to find out what caused my psychosis. It is believed that both genetic and environmental factors play a role [11].

My nan had experienced hallucinations, when she was nearly ninety, mind you. She had got ill before moving into a nursing home. At one stage in front of the doctor she told him she could see a knight on a white horse on the roof of the bungalow opposite. Later she saw water running down the walls and the gaps in the pavement opening up. My other nan wasn't happy unless she was worrying about something, she also had OCD when leaving the house. I remember sitting in the car waiting for her to do all her checks. My twin sister had not suffered psychosis or OCD so it couldn't all be down to genetic make-up.

My memory and anxiety levels remain affected, so my cortisol levels could have been very high before my breakdown. Sleep deprivation, caffeine and alcohol all increase cortisol [1]. I had been suffering sleep deprivation and had consumed a large amount of caffeine before my breakdown which can't have helped. My husband had found bottles of Coke littering the kitchen. I'd had a false memory that the Coke had been taken and tested to see if it had been spiked. It is quite ironic that the seemingly harmless caffeine may have worsened my condition.

The molecule of cortisol is shown on the next page. Surely it couldn't be that harmful consisting of only hydrogen, carbon and oxygen! It's a hormone meaning it carries chemical signals around our bodies in the blood. The release of cortisol is controlled by another hormone released from the pituitary gland at the base of the brain. Target cells and organs respond to cortisol. It has many effects but I am most interested in those on the brain.

The molecule
Cortisol [1]

The area of the brain (hippocampus – who came up with that name?!) that is responsible for memories has many cortisol receptors. This means that the cells here respond to cortisol. The receptors within the cells get overloaded and they literally die from excitement. So with really high levels degeneration can happen; apparently this can be reversible, which is a relief. Although there is a hint that chronic stress can cause brain aging [24]. Basically your brain is made up of nerve cells and the connections between these form when memories are made. If cells degenerate these memories are lost. I was now having problems remembering whether I'd taken my tablets during the day. I'm going to invest in one of those containers you can buy. Older people normally have them!

Circadian rhythm has an effect on cortisol in our bodies and this explains why I'm reaching for an anxiety tablet before I've even left the house. It reaches a max after waking up. This is deliberate apparently to help you feel more alert. Levels are then supposed to fall until you are all relaxed and ready to sleep. It would have been interesting to see what my levels were like over the previous few years. The amygdala, an area of the brain responsible for feelings of fear, is increased in size and activity by cortisol explaining my feelings of anxiety [14].

Currently I'd do things to try and deal with this evil molecule cortisol which had to be balanced. Hormones are an essential part of life they help us develop and control many mechanisms but they do have to be balanced. I'd come back from work and then walk into town rather than drive. Surely that was enough exercise? I'd avoid stressful circumstances. My husband referred to it as me acquiescing. But there was no arguing with some people and it was bad for my health. However, considering all this the stress response has evolved for a reason.

Cortisol and adrenaline (another hormone) would prepare the body for action. Cortisol would ensure the release of glucose to be used by body cells and adrenaline would among other things increase heart rate pumping blood round in a more urgent manner.

The whole stressful situation causes a fight or flight mechanism. For instance, once at work I would sometimes find the urge to leave and go home. I never really felt the urge to fight which is probably good in my position! Maybe I should invest in a punch bag. Both the hormones adrenaline and cortisol increase during fight or flight and if physical release of flight or fight doesn't happen cortisol can build up in your blood. You need some way of getting cortisol back to normal levels [33].

So what was triggering my anxious feelings that would play havoc with my hormones?

What someone says	How it makes me feel
'Sorry, Sam. I've had to use you for cover'	Until recently this made me anxious. Oh my God what are the classes going to be like? Will I know their names?
'Mum, where did I put my bus pass?'	Guilty. It was 'wear what you like day' and I should have known his bus pass was in his blazer so he might forget it.
'You could take the big car.'	Anxious. Rather not thank you, how am I supposed to park that? What about the narrow country lanes?
'You could come on the back of my Guzzi.'	Anxious. I had a motorbike licence and had enjoyed riding them in the past. Dad's motorbike skills were good, it was the other people on the roads that worried me.
'Mum, come here, he's all red and sunburnt!'	Guilty. It was the second day of our Portugal holiday and the day had been cloudy but both boys had got mild sunburn as we thought they wouldn't burn. The risks of such mistakes were well known especially now with Google.

These are just examples. Anxiety and guilt are closely linked and I would often blame myself for bad things that happened [13]. Some things I just needed to move on from but would sometimes let them eat away at me inside. I remember someone I used to work with saying that being a parent brought with it feelings of guilt. In recent years my main guilt came from working so hard on teaching and not spending as much time as I should with my family and friends.

This website highlights the problem of negative thinking:
http://www.anxietyspecialist.co.uk/Anxiety-Bristol-Bath.html

I'd been told again today by my husband to watch my negative feelings especially about work and to not talk negatively about work in front of the kids. I found this hard as I was honest about my feelings, but someone at work had said her sons had worried about her when she worked. I'd have to find new ways of venting about the pressure I felt at work. I'd aim to take control of these feelings as lack of control can cause anxiety.

These feelings were no doubt triggering the release of cortisol and I'd have to watch this. Maybe it was a case of balancing my negative thoughts and feelings like balancing my hormones. After watching various science based programmes I was aware that there were scientific reasons not to be anxious about minor everyday things.

After all, I have no control over the following:

The sun is limited and one day it will engulf the Earth. (It is in its stable part of its life at the moment but will become a red giant.)
The moon is moving away from the Earth and this will affect our magnetic field and Earth's spin.
Aliens could be out there and they may not be friendly.
A super volcano may erupt in Yellowstone Park any day now.
A disease could wipe out everyone on the planet.

Maybe such thoughts and a defeatist attitude that 'we were all doomed anyway' weren't that useful and maybe technology would advance enough to allow some of us to escape at least. The nurses in Sapphire Ward had told me to concentrate on positive thoughts after all. So the sun is limited but we've got another few billion years yet! Again it would take over a billion years for the moon to move away far enough to destabilize the Earth or make it uninhabitable. Maybe I've been watching too much *X-files* lately so thoughts of aliens popped up. As for a super volcano eruption there is very little you can do about that apart from evacuate and conserve supplies. But apparently there is a one in 700,000 annual chance of a volcanic eruption at the site [10]. That's a small chance and surely some countries would survive. As for the last one my eldest son plays this game on his tablet where you come up with a disease and try to wipe out the world. Even he hasn't managed to wipe out the world and so maybe we're safe; I think the game is called Pandemic II.

I had just been doing some internet shopping and treated myself to a little notepad of positive thoughts one for each day. When it arrived I was a little disappointed as it was only one thought per month.

I liked the 'create your own sunshine' one. Follow your dreams wasn't so good as most of my dreams were nightmares.

Well at least my dreams had started to stabilise, three months after my failed attempt to come off my tablets. I still dreamt but they weren't as vivid and disturbing. I've heard that dreams are a way your brain recovers from the day's events. Anxious people had more information from the day to sort because they were in a heightened alert state. Most websites had meanings for a dream involving a boat sinking but not of a boat shrinking surprisingly enough. But according to the website dreambible.com a dream about a boat signified how you were dealing with negative emotions. The huge waves I had seen signified uncertainty. At the time of the dream it was never certain what I would face at work so maybe there was more to this dream analysing malarkey then some people thought. Dreams occur during rapid eye movement (REM). Scientists have learned to identify what we dream about by the signals seen in the brain [29]. I could imagine vivid dreams would cause more of a signal.

What about the things that I had seen so clearly when I was awake that had not actually been there? Looking at the types of psychosis I decided I had suffered a brief psychotic episode [8], for which relapses are quite common [17]. I had suffered delusions (thinking I was involved in a big plot) and hallucinations (seeing people from work when they weren't actually there). During my relapse I had gone in to shut down which may have been catatonic behaviour. These symptoms are described on the web [17]. I don't think I suffered disorganised speech, what I was saying was clear it just didn't make a lot of sense. With so many possible symptoms and the fact that everyone has different levels of these must make it very hard for mental health nurses and doctors.

'Caffeine can cause hallucinations' [16]. But how many caffeinated drinks would you need to cause these? Just how much had I consumed in the days leading up to my breakdown? I don't remember. Looking for other possible reasons, not enough stimulation can cause hallucinations but in my case too much stimulation, as I was in a high emotional state [15]. Auditory and visual hallucinogens can come about when we imagine things so clearly and the brain cannot determine that we have in fact generated these sights and sounds ourselves. This is due to brain connectivity problems and telling the difference between self-produced and external stimuli [32]. I've always had a good imagination and during my illness this was very powerful.

So why did it happen to me? You can work out the likelihood of being ill from stress factors looking at the list supplied by mind tools based on the Holmes and Rahe Stress Scale [31]. I scored 107 before my breakdown. Apparently I had had only a low to moderate chance of becoming ill in the near future. Yet I had got spectacularly ill in what to me was a very short amount of time.

The factors which I had identified were:

Business readjustment (contracts introduced)

Change in responsibilities at work (I was writing a course)

Trouble with boss (I wasn't really in trouble but I had pointed out the contracts were incorrect to my principal)

Change in sleeping habits (I had not slept well leading up to the breakdown, waking up early and discussing my problems with my husband, almost discussing who had the most stressful job and why!)

Reading the other stress events I was glad I hadn't

suffered these. I knew other people who had suffered; for example, the loss of a spouse or had gone through a separation yet they had coped better than me. I know it's not on the same emotional scale but maybe training to teach should be up there with the big ones. Seven in every ten teachers and lecturers said their health had suffered because of the job [35]. After all, teaching takes over your mind. If you are not taking lessons you are planning them, which can be an endless task, marking work, reporting grades and behaviour and more. This is a recent quote about a science teacher who had recently killed herself: 'Her mind was in overdrive she couldn't rest and there were times she was unable to concentrate' [9].

Health discussions would sometimes come up at work. A colleague said she had watched four Harry Potter movies over the weekend. So she hadn't done much preparation. I told her it had to be done sometimes and your mind worked better after rest. Recently two of us got the lurgy but managed to soldier on. I'd feel like death but paced myself as much as possible. I'd tell the students that we were going to talk about infectious diseases that morning. I could then relate to how I had got the virus from breathing droplets in the air and talk about gross diseases. But seriously, sickness was rife in the school and staff turnaround was high. I said, 'The kids are making us ill!' It has been shown that stress does affect the immune system. Cortisol and corticosteroids suppress lymphocytes [27]. Lymphocytes are key players in the response to foreign bodies such as pathogens in our bodies. They are super hero cells they produce antibodies which are used against specific unwanted invaders in our bodies. Cortisol affects the number of white blood cells or lymphocytes and how they function [26]. I had given in and had a few days off sick, I just felt so tired and dozy and a chest infection had started. To add to it all I had a cold sore which was trying to take over my face. It was only the second time I'd been off sick since I started but I still worried about the return to work interview. The kids at work had been remarkably tactful about my cold sore. I looked at the triggers for getting these and basically it was because I was run down. It was actually costing the government not to tackle stress and fatigue. One day someone would realise. It seemed particularly bad in schools.

Walking into town with my cold sore that was now a big scab didn't do much for my paranoia. I'd put some make-up on but who was I kidding? As a group of people walked towards me I'd casually look away. A couple of them laughed but it wasn't about me, they were just having a good time. In a way I wished I'd waited until it was dark. I managed to get into the Co-op without many people noticing me. I saw someone from work and said, 'Look what happened to me,' pointing to my lip. She smiled and asked if I was feeling better.

Shortly after this when I was checking out the plasters, the fire alarm started. Seriously, what was it with me and fire alarms? The manager came out and said we'd all have to leave the store. Not like when we were in Sapphire Ward when we just got moved to a different area, they didn't want us running off I guess. I waited a little while outside, in the end I had to brave another shop to get some much needed supplies. My hubby was at work and he wasn't feeling great either. When I got back, I googled about cold sores, probably should have done that when I was younger.

I'd first got them when I was about eight. My anxiety went up a little as I read that it could be spread to the eyes and you could get scarring on the eye. I tried to put this from my mind and reminded myself that I'd taken care not to spread it. My son and I decided we'd look at pictures of cold sores on Google. Boy, was that bad! Only about four of the pictures were worse than mine. The next day I was no better so I donned a plaster and got myself to the doctor. I made an appointment and was prescribed yet more tablets; antibiotics and antivirals. I think I had got quite run down. Now I was to be on seventeen tablets in one day for a while. That would test my memory. Was this the way of the modern world to overwork and stress people so they started to rattle when they walked? Maybe more people should be tested for cortisol levels and given some down time if needed. I'm not asking for a lot, just a duvet day like you get in America.

No, seriously, we all need to be careful, although some people seem to cope better than others. If you have been stressed for a long period your feedback mechanism between your brain and the adrenal glands can go wrong and levels may rocket [28]. This whole research thing has been a wake-up call to me as my tablets do not tackle cortisol so I will need to try and lower my levels by:

1) Avoiding caffeine. This would be hard as it is what I looked forward to during breaks at work and when I got to work. Drinking decaf coffee was much like drinking non-alcoholic beer, not very satisfying. Maybe I could just moderate my numbers of caffeinated drinks especially if I felt stressed.

2) Avoiding alcohol. Well, I had managed this lately as antibiotics do not mix with beer. Those tempting craft beers would have to wait. Alcohol also weakens the immune system – note to self at this point. Why had I started having a drink each evening? I had used work as an excuse, it was a hard school to work in but I needed better ways of unwinding that would fit in with a busy evening at home. My hubby had set up a turbo trainer but I never seemed in the mood for that. If work makes you feel like drink in the evening with more at weekends maybe it was time to change jobs again. My mentality had become 'I'd survived the day so I deserved a beer'.

3) Exercising more. This was a vital part of fight or flight which lowered stress hormones. This would be a toughie working full-time with dark evenings and things to do at the weekend. I couldn't do that now with a chest infection but would schedule it in somehow. I had tried exercising just before my breakdown. I had gone out jogging but it was clearly too little too late. I'd not been jogging for months

now. It was all very well the government recommending regular exercise but would they tackle lack of time and resources. Would time be allowed at the end of the school/work day for people to use onsite gyms? I doubt it.

4) Reduce and manage stress. I'd started to learn not to take work life too seriously and to treat it more as day by day. Health had to take priority and I now knew this.

5) Sleep well. This hadn't been a problem lately and I'd continue to go to bed by 9.30!

6) Oh I like this one, been meaning to get a cat for ages. Stroking one reduces cortisol levels [4].

Reading this article about cats is when I found out about the goody hormone oxytocin. Another article said I needed to increase this by hugs, laughing, playing and romance [22]. It also says to smile more, most people at work know I'm a smiley person even in the face of adversity, as for romance I was going to have to spend more time on that. Difficult I guess when your husband works shifts and you're in bed by 9.30. There are quizzes on line about oxytocin levels; the questions are quite personal if you get my drift. Basically, it's all about quality time with the people you love. May be this family holiday was long overdue.

So how else can I lower cortisol naturally? Laughter is a good way. Recently I had braved another trip to a comedy club. My fears had been allayed when we had arrived and the seats we had were stools upstairs, the one I was on was behind a pillar. We were pretty safe there as we couldn't really be seen from the stage. It was a good evening but to be honest we had more fun trying to take selfies of ourselves outside the theatre. My friend is confident to say the least. She asked some passers-by to take our photo but we still weren't pleased with the results and had a laugh.

The fact that you need laughter is probably why you need a good sense of humour to survive in stressful jobs. Even the thought of laughing has been shown to reduce stress hormones [19]. All these natural ways to help control cortisol were good, even though I'd worked in the pharmaceutical industry for eleven years I thought that natural was better where possible!

Laughing also works by increasing oxytocin levels. The more I hear about oxytocin the more I like it. Its chemical structure is more complex than that of cortisol but it is similar in that it is characterised by carbon rings. I'm not sure how it does it but it reduces cortisol levels. This time the bigger molecule wins and size really does matter in the battle of the hormones.

Still, at least my recent wait at the doctors gave me chance to read up about my anxiety tablets. Seems I should take more note as to whether I've taken them or not as a too higher dose or stopping them suddenly can cause a heart attack. I knew there were side effects of my medicine but had tried life without them and figured a low dose which controlled my anxiety and psychosis was probably best. Basically propranolol is a beta blocker. You may have heard these take action on the heart. Beta receptors are found around the heart and normally they will respond to adrenaline causing the heart to beat faster. The beta blockers combine with the receptors so adrenaline can't. When we get anxious, our heart rate and blood pressure go up so beta blockers help reduce this. But what if I was faced with a real life tiger situation, would I be able to respond quickly enough? Maybe I'll be able to think about what action I take more clearly, having read the how to survive a tiger attack tips [23] I think I'll be fine.

They are:

Method 1: Try to remain calm and back away slowly. Think that would be easier on my tablets.

Method 2: Make yourself look big. That's got to take guts too.

Method 3: Repel an attacking tiger with noise. Interestingly it says here to if you have a firearm, fire it into the air. Think I would actually fire it at the tiger especially if it's running at me! Surely my steady hand due to my anxiety tablets would help.

Method 4: Do whatever you can to survive. Don't worry, I'll do that.

Apparently running away isn't any good, well unless you can get into a car or something. Then I might need my extra heart rate.

How about the other tablets which I had tried to come off in the summer? These were olanzapine. There are a lot of negative forums about this drug and it's true there were possible side effects and it was hard to give up. But how was it chemically helping me? Well it is used to treat hallucinations and delusions. I haven't had these since my relapse in 2012. Interestingly, tremor is a side effect of olanzapine but I've always had a slight tremor [18]. Olanzapine levels can drop on antiviral drugs so I'll keep an eye on that.

Taking that many tablets in a day was bound to cause some interaction. I don't really like to call it antipsychotic but that's what they are. Basically psychotic illness is considered to be caused by disturbances in the activity of neurotransmitters (mainly dopamine) in the brain [20]. Neurotransmitters are chemicals that pass between nerve cells so that an electrical impulse can be triggered in the receiving cell and the message carried forward. Olanzapine is another type of blocker; this time it blocks receptors that respond to dopamine. I knew that somehow the small dose I was on was stabilizing me mentally and for now that was enough to keep me on them.

Like cortisol, dopamine can affect health if in high amounts; its release during stress is linked to cortisol [33]. Dopamine is not only released during stress it is also released during pleasurable experiences. Many addictive drugs can cause psychotic episodes linked to dopamine levels [21]. After reading the long list of drugs that cause psychotic episodes I'm not surprised the staff at the Ward kept asking my husband if I'd taken drugs. I'd never taken any; my vices were alcohol and caffeine. For me my cause was stress and lack of sleep. My dopamine levels had probably rocketed; this affects specific pathways in the brain. It is released in times of stress into the prefrontal cortex part of the brain [5]. For example, the pathway for self-generated thoughts and reality could have been affected causing my hallucinations. Memory is also affected [5] explaining why (during my stay in hospital) I couldn't remember what job my husband did, emotion explaining why I was all over the place and delusions explaining some of my bizarre behaviour such as dancing and trying to open doors in hospital. Indeed I did have many of the symptoms found to come from too higher levels of dopamine [2]. Interestingly feelings of suspicion are one of them and I had been very suspicious of people around me, for example when they asked to see my children's photos. Dopamine is needed in a balanced amount again. Not enough of it had been linked with depression [7] so I now know why the doctor later advised that I get out and do things that I enjoyed after not coping with my return to work. But too much dopamine was equally catastrophic.

My other symptoms like blurred vision and chest pains had been mild and short lived but I will keep an eye out for these in the future. Elevated adrenaline levels can put pressure on the eyes sometimes resulting in blurred vision [12]. Chest pains can result from how your breathing changes when you are anxious, it was learning to recognise your breathing has changed which would help. I was able to concentrate on my breathing easily when doing a wordsearch that I had recently loaded on to my Kindle. But I couldn't just whip this out whenever I felt the need.

So what were my anxiety levels like now? I used a questionnaire on the net to find out. I came out at 60% and healthy levels are less than 40% [34]. I know questionnaires aren't seen as wholly scientific but for how you feel, which affects the chemicals inside your body, can only really be assessed by asking questions about how you feel.

My score for OCD was quite low which I was pleased about as this can also become a big problem for people leading to further anxiety. My anxiety level had been a bit high even while off work sick I was experiencing flash forwards about my holiday to Thailand as it approached, mainly about losing each other in the crowds. I'd bought a map book but that had only shown how big Bangkok was. I'd have positive feelings and imagined swimming on a glorious beach, the boys with UV swim tops on!

The whole chest infection problem had made me anxious as it was taking ages to clear up, after my hubby's bad infection this year I knew how dangerous they could get. Eventually the antibiotics started to kick in. I was annoyed with myself for not taking it easier when the warning signs were there. I felt really tired at work before the virus hit over two weeks ago but it was hard at work at the moment. A recent inspection, for which I'm glad I slept through as I was signed off work, had deemed the school needed to improve for teaching and learning. The biggest barrier it seemed to me was the attitude and behaviour of many of the students and unfortunately this did not seem to really be improving.

I recently went in with the notorious class after they had to be split up in a previous lesson to try and subdue them. When I was in with them it took thirty minutes for them to settle. Although they were better this time as the new behaviour expert had started teaching them and I was covering one of his lessons. He'd had a word with them before I faced them. He seemed to have the energy and confidence to tackle that group which for a lot of us had quite frankly been zapped. Some of the Year 11 students referred to him as the Defence Against the Dark Arts teacher as this teacher also changed yearly in Harry Potter. It was true two other behaviour experts had been in for the previous two years and left. One of them even had army training yet had still been unable to make a difference. We could do with this new one sticking around as he himself had estimated it would take maybe five years to get behaviour to a workable level. I asked who they thought I was like out of Harry Potter and we all agreed, Sybill Trelawney. Maybe it was her slight madness in manner, as I didn't walk round with a crystal ball. I hope it wasn't her incompetence!

Out of the classroom, behaviour was also still a problem. Yesterday, a student had kicked a double door open right in front of me and another student had squared up to the teacher and swore at her because she had confiscated his phone. It almost seemed the norm for this to happen, so at least now I didn't get anxious about it. I'd been through a lot in the past few years and was wary of getting that ill again.

So what conclusions could I come to after writing this book? Who were the real goodies and baddies in my story?

It was not in fact the people from work that I had grouped into goodies and baddies and that I had seen in my conspiracy theory. It was the chemicals within my body. I had been right to say that anxiety was running through my veins. Cortisol and then dopamine in excess levels were the baddies showing the danger of chronic stress to long term health. The goodies may be oxytocin to combat cortisol and the changes that I make with help, to my lifestyle. Changing jobs just over two years ago had seemed like a good idea but my new role had different stresses largely due to the behaviour of the students and the pressure I felt to help out. Other more successful changes may come in the form of a cat called Kitty that we would rescue after the holiday, an exercise regime of some sort (got to do something!) and quality time. Some way I'll find space for these in my home and work schedule, teachers had even less time for this due to constant planning and other duties.

Reading a recent ATL report [36] there was a need for happiness and mental health to be looked at for education staff alongside that of the children and young people in their care. I find if I'm happier and less stressed I enjoy my lessons and the students seem to respond better which makes me even happier. There is so much to tackle in education and we are seriously behind other countries in wellbeing. Yep it's going to take money, resources and time.

Let's avoid this vicious cycle of pressure, stress and then illness (mental and physical) that's affected me and so many others.

Epilogue

It has taken me quite a lot of strength to read this through again. I think it's a complete enough picture. Hopefully it will help many people with mental health problems in the future either directly or through those that help them. I was lucky enough to have a good support network of family and friends; some people aren't so lucky.

Mental health problems can be invisible or appear bizarre and can take on many forms. Don't be afraid to talk about your feelings and ask for help or to ask someone how they are, or if you can help them. If someone you know may be severely stressed at work try to persuade them to get to the doctors and to have some rest. Think about the dangers that may unfold. This is my legacy that I intend to carry on.

…And by the way, we made it to Thailand and back, and it was amazing. It was straightforward getting to the airport hotel and we relaxed there before heading off to the terminal in the morning. The freezing fog cleared and our flight wasn't delayed by much. When we did board, the boys were impressed with the gadgets on the plane. Every seat had a screen. One channel was a camera fitted on the outside of the plane. I didn't mind watching this during taxiing and take-off. But once we were in the air I couldn't help feeling anxious. Negative thoughts crept into my mind. I told my youngest son to switch over. He must have been a bit anxious during take-off as he had reached over and grabbed my hand. Seeing the plane on screen in the air I thought there were hundreds of ways we could fall out of the sky. I didn't want to see any problems unfold. Incoming torpedoes and engine fire were just some silly scenarios that came to mind. The only one I admitted to thinking of was a possible bird strike. Thankfully the plane journey was uneventful apart from spilling some wine down my leg and bag!

We finally got through immigration and after accidently picking up the wrong suitcase and realising just in time we walked out to meet our Thai relatives and my father-in-law. It was great to see them again. I hadn't seen my half brother-in-law since he was twelve or thirteen and he was now twenty-five!

Over the holiday I relaxed and I would go near to say I had become cured. OK, I was still on my tablets but I felt good. We were made to feel so welcome. The Thai people were so smiley, Thailand is called the land of the smiles. They were constantly snacking which I could also relate to.

A lot of the stress had been taken away from the holiday as our hosts spoke the lingo and held the boys' arms as we crossed the roads. My step brother-in law was a skilled driver and negotiated the busy roads in our twelve-seater, making it look easy. We were grateful he could make both of our big road trips. In fact I only had a couple of anxious moments during our stay.

We'd had sticky rice in bamboo pots. Only they had been wrapped like a present. I'd got the package open but halfway down mine I had a pain in my teeth. I put my finger in my mouth and found a staple. I knew it was good to have a staple diet but not literally! I'd started to think maybe I'd swallowed one or the boys had. Surely we would have noticed as it squeezed past our epiglottis. What if it had got lodged somewhere in our long digestive tract or scraped along our soft tissue? This was not the way to get your stomach stapled. Luckily some reassuring thoughts arrived. I remember seeing on TV once this man that ate glass and metal and came to no harm. I think he actually enjoyed it.

Another anxious moment was minor; this was that I had possibly stained the hire car seat with sun tan lotion, well I had smothered the boys in it. I was determined to not let them burn. They didn't and we had enjoyed a few lovely mornings playing on the beach.

Grandpa had talked about his time on the submarine. I had thought how submariners coped being in a tin can a bit like a plane but this time under metres of water with again little chance of survival if something went wrong. At least with my work I wasn't risking my life in such a direct way.

For the second beach trip we had seen a jellyfish and I was impressed by how calm I had been about this. I had not identified it as a box jellyfish and could see no others in the water. With anxiety and medication there is a balance between being over anxious and freezing unable to do anything in difficult situations or being over calm and almost complacent but able to think logically.

Thanks to my pills and new attitude I had also calmly dealt with suspected deep vein thrombosis in my right leg halfway through the flight on the way home, my eldest sniffing insect repellent in the car and feeling numb in the legs and my youngest throwing up and going green after eating a nut of similar colour.

On one of our road trips we had stopped at a service station and I had negotiated the 'stand and crouch' toilets. I'm not sure how the elderly faired. As I came out the others were looking at a music stall. Folk music, which I hated, was quite big in Thailand. I found a disco one for my step brother-in-law. It had the Bee Gees and Abba on. He got the lady to play it. 'Staying Alive' came on and I started to dance spontaneously. I felt the happiest I'd felt in ages. I think I had embarrassed my boys though! Our driver clearly liked the new music and tapped the steering wheel to the beat. Again this made me happy. Finding the time to be happy would be my new motto.

So there it is; my dad said I should end on a positive note. I was beating anxiety, and writing this book had helped. Despite all the possibilities the only real harm that we had come to on holiday was when I'd fallen flat on my face at a waterfall on slippery rocks. A group of Thai people were behind me. In true character they showed genuine concern and didn't smirk. One said in perfect English, 'Are you OK?' She then held out her hand for me to step across a rock. I'd suffered only minor bruises, it was time to start living again.

References

1) http://dujs.dartmouth.edu/2011/02/the-physiology-of-stress-cortisol-and-the-hypothalamic-pituitary-adrenal-axis/#.WDSCcrKLR0w

2) http://mentalhealthdaily.com/2015/04/01/high-dopamine-levels-symptoms-adverse-reactions/

3) http://onlinelibrary.wiley.com/doi/10.1111/pcn.12259/pdf

4) http://pets.thenest.com/can-stroking-cats-fur-relieve-stress-8220.html

5) http://scicurious.scientopia.org/2012/12/05/stressed-out-and-not-thinking-straight-blame-the-dopamine-in-your-prefrontal-cortex/

6) http://www.anxietyspecialist.co.uk/Anxiety-Bristol-Bath.html

7) http://www.balancingbrainchemistry.co.uk/peter-smith/38/Dopamine-Deficient-Depression.html

8) http://www.camh.ca/en/hospital/health_information/a_z_mental_health_and_addiction_information/psychosis/first_episode_psychosis_information_guide/Pages/fep_types.aspx

9) http://www.dailymail.co.uk/news/article-3925256/Newly-promoted-science-teacher-threw-motorway-viaduct-swamped-work-sleeping-three-hours-night.html

10) http://www.dailymail.co.uk/sciencetech/article-3189619/What-happen-Yellowstone-s-supervolcano-erupted-Experts-warn-90-000-immediate-deaths-nuclear-winter-US.html

11) http://www.earlypsychosis.ca/pages/diagnosed/what-causes-psychosis

12) http://www.healthcentral.com/anxiety/c/4182/151322/anxiety-problems/

13) http://www.healthcentral.com/anxiety/c/8468/21164/anxiety-guilt/

14) http://www.huffingtonpost.com/2014/11/18/brain-stress_n_6148470.html

15) http://www.humanillnesses.com/Behavioral-Health-Fe-Mu/Hallucination.html

16) http://www.livescience.com/3230-caffeine-hallucinations.html

17) http://www.msdmanuals.com/professional/psychiatric-disorders/schizophrenia-and-related-disorders/brief-psychotic-disorder.

18) http://www.namihelps.org/assets/PDFs/fact-sheets/Medications/Zyprexa.pdf

19) http://www.nature.com/news/2008/080407/full/news.2008.741.html

20) http://www.netdoctor.co.uk/medicines/brain-and-nervous-system/a7807/zyprexa-olanzapine/

21) http://www.nhs.uk/Conditions/Psychosis/Pages/Causes.aspx

22) http://www.saragottfriedmd.com/why-do-i-feel-disconnected-the-cortisol-oxytocin-connection/

23) http://www.wikihow.com/Survive-a-Tiger-Attack

24) http://www.youramazingbrain.org/brainchanges/stressbrain.htm

25) http://www.yourhormones.info/Hormones/Cortisol.aspx

26) https://adrenalfatigue.org/ the-anti-inflammatory-effects-of-cortisol/

27) https://adrenalfatiguesolution.com/stress-immune-system/

28) https://breakingmuscle.com/learn/the-ups-and-downs-of-cortisol-what-you-need-to-know

29) https://mic.com/articles/90973/the-fascinating-science-of-what-dreaming-does-to-your-brain#.r5Pd16DsE

30) https://www.cogneurosociety.org/cortisol_memory

31) https://www.mindtools.com/pages/article/newTCS_82.htm

32) https://www.ncbi.nlm.nih.gov/pmc/articles/PMC2702442/

33) https://www.psychologytoday.com/blog/the-athletes-way/201301/cortisol-why-the-stress-hormone-is-public-enemy-no-1 (web page description)

34) https://www.recoveryformula.com/quiz/start

35) https://www.theguardian.com/education/2008/aug/31/teaching.teachersworkload

36) Report The Magazine from ATL, The Education Union November/December 2016. Page 15.

30568461R00056

Printed in Great Britain
by Amazon